Walking For Weight Loss:

Get In Shape, Feel Confident And Be Healthier For Life

Andy Johnson

Table of Contents

Introduction

I want to thank you and congratulate you for downloading the book, "Walking for Weight Loss".

Want to walk but don't know how to start? Want to lose weight, but don't know which way is right? Well in that case, this is the book for you!

Walking for Weight Loss will take you step by step, and show you the advantages of walking.

One of the biggest stigmas in the health and fitness world is that you need to be a jogger to be able to live a healthy lifestyle. Often this stigma includes getting up at dawn or just before dawn to jog the neighborhood, then you come home, shower, and then begin the rest of your day.

While this works for some people, it doesn't work for everyone. The older you get, the more exponentially difficult it becomes to jog in general much less every day, and jogging is particularly hard on those with arthritis, bad knees, back problems, and a number of other additional circumstances.

Does that mean that if you're older or if you have bad knees that you shouldn't even exercise? Absolutely not! In fact, a few studies have come out in recent years arguing that daily walkers are much healthier in the long term than joggers are because walking daily is kinder on your joints and skeletal system, and a well-paced walker often has an easier time toning muscles as the walker has more flexibility to focus on muscle groups as opposed to getting into a jogging rhythm and working the same muscle groups.

Additionally, several physicians have recently found that walkers (opposed to joggers) have lower blood pressure. While it's important to elevate your heart rate while walking to achieve the desired outcome (fitness, toning, and potential weight loss), physicians have argued that walking instead of jogging keeps the heart rate steady at a lower pace and thus helps to lower blood pressure without taxing the cardiac muscles too much.

If you want to learn more about these and other health benefits associated with walking for weight loss and walking for overall health, take a look.

information is without contract or any type of guarantee assurance.

The trademarks that are used are without any consent, and the publication of the trademark is without permission or backing by the trademark owner. All trademarks and brands within this book are for clarifying purposes only and are the owned by the owners themselves, not affiliated with this document.

Chapter 1:
Walk For Confidence

Walking is easy. Most of us do it every day, sometimes without even thinking about it. If you are fortunate not to have any health problems, you may find yourself as a busy professional who knows the quickest route to drive somewhere, and always looks for the first row parking spot. Can you walk? Yes, but you don't have time. You are a professional, and you have responsibilities.

If you are retired, you work from home, or if you are a stay at home parent, you may find that you have time to walk on some days, but don't have time to walk on other days. It's hard to know what your day is going to look like when it begins, and sometimes you are hesitant to commit to anything that you know you won't be able to keep up. You don't have a gym membership, you don't make plans more than one day out, or maybe you find joy and freedom in making plans impulsively.

Maybe you just have low-self-esteem right now. Maybe you're grieving, maybe you're at a rough patch in your life, maybe you're unemployed, or you're a little more overweight than you thought you were. Maybe you realize that a change needs to happen, but you're so comfortable in the life you have that you're afraid of being shot down again. You don't have the energy to try something new. You want change, but you don't know how to make it.

Would you believe that walking will boost your confidence, irrespective of whatever lifestyle you adopt?

Why do you think that elementary school students have recess every day? Yes, on the surface it's because they're highly energetic children who need time to run around and get a little tired so that they can sit in their chairs again, but any teacher will tell you that even the best students learn better if they get up and move around between long periods of study.

Let's take this concept to adults: you could be a professional, but that doesn't mean that you're confident —and you may very well be confident, but it's likely that being a professional means that you're stressed out about work often as well.

By getting into the habit of going for a walk every day at a time of your choosing (most professionals enjoy a walk first thing in the morning, but based on your work or what time you get off you may find that walking when you get home at the end of the day is suitable as well) will relax you and ground you more.

By managing something easy like walking, you are in control, you are responsible, and you are taking initiative to do something good for yourself. That's confidence.

If you're retired, work from home, or a stay at home parent, this concept is no different. Sometimes you don't know what your day is going to be like because you a lot of other factors monopolize your schedule.

If you commit to walking daily or every other day in a block of time that is untouched by other things, you will find yourself more confident because you are in control of something. This doesn't mean that the other things in your life are bad or that they need to stop. However, by adding something for you and only for you that you can control will breed confidence.

If you are going through a rough patch in your life and you know you need to make a change but don't know what it is, go for a walk around the block. The fresh air will be good, the circulation will be good, and you don't have to be gone a long time. Fresh air is the lifeblood of circulation, and circulation helps things to move. In your case, they could move you from this place you find yourself in.

Confidence is having control, and walking is an easily controlled, healthy activity. You can walk around the block or you can walk a 3 mile hiking trail—it doesn't matter. You are in control; it is up to you how, where, and for how long you want to walk.

Application:

What is an area of your schedule that you can control? You don't have to commit to it yet, just jot a few ideas down in a journal. Next, write about how you would feel if you have one small area of your life that you could control, and how you would feel if this small thing could also provide health benefits, make you feel better, and potentially help you lose weight.

Chapter 2:
Health Advantages Of Walking

There are a number of health advantages to walking regularly.

On the surface, it seems that the only benefits are control, confidence, and peace of mind. These are very strong and important benefits (and later we'll see why these are more important than we think they are). If you have control, confidence, and peace of mind, walking helps to improve your daily life. The rest of your personal or professional schedule may not change, but at least if you have control over one activity that is just yours, you may find that you have peace of mind over those other daily duties.

It's often recommended that widows or widowers get a dog after a spouse has passed away. While it seems like a difficult responsibility to take care of something else when you need taking care of yourself, physicians have found that widows and widowers who follow this instruction are less despondent not only because he or she is taking care of something that will love him/her unconditionally, but also the widow or widower now has the responsibility of taking that dog for daily or twice-daily walks.

Walking the dog gets the bereaved spouse out of the house, out into fresh air, meeting neighbors, having companionship, and controlling at least one small aspect of his or her life.

Your mindset is everything to your health. Once you start recognizing confidence, responsibility, and peace of mind over this easy, small thing that you can control, physicians have found that walkers have lower blood pressure. Why? To some, it's because stress has been reduced through an outlet. To others it's an exercise. However, walking provides peace of mind to everyone who practices it.

Other health benefits of walking regularly include muscle toning. Because you're walking at a regular, slower pace than, say, jogging, you have the flexibility to work with different muscle groups. Some walkers will walk on their toes for a brief while to stretch out their hamstrings, some walkers bend their knees more to work out their calves more, some walkers take extra large steps occasionally as if lunging, and some walkers will start out at a slow pace, escalate to a fast pace, and then decelerate back to a slow pace before arriving at his or her home.

But whether you actively work on muscle toning or not, walking regularly is an effective aid to weight loss. In recent years, doctors have found that more patients who walk regularly lose more weight than patients who jog. The reason for this is because walking is gentler on your system (particularly on your joints, your skeletal system, and your back) so walkers have the ability to walk longer more regularly than joggers who might take the day off because of joint pain. Walkers generally have more endurance than some joggers and stay active and healthy longer into their life than joggers who quit when they get "too old" or have too many extenuating circumstances. Walking is easy, and for some it's easy to commit to daily or every other day.

Walking is the safest form of exercise, so it is ideal for everyone no matter what body type or age they are. While walking doesn't cause weight loss overnight, if you walk 15-20 minutes 3-5 times a week, you'll lose about half a pound to a pound a week. While this doesn't sound like a lot, keeping this regimen up for 20 weeks results in weight loss up to 20 lbs.

The average amount of weight loss per person varies for however many minutes they walk. However, the more you weigh the more calories you burn during a 15-20 minute walk. This is particularly beneficial for those who might think they're too overweight to start a workout regimen: the heavier you are, the more walking will help you lose weight. The more weight you lose, the more confident you will feel, and the healthier you will be.

Application:

The next time you go for a walk, bring a watch or some kind of time piece (If you have a smart phone, it may be helpful to set a timer or to set a stopwatch). Explore the block in your neighborhood and see what route you can comfortably take that will last 15-20 minutes. You may find that walking in your neighborhood is more convenient for you than going to the gym, but if you're more comfortable going to the gym, get in the habit of walking 15-20 minutes on the treadmill before or after your workout.

Chapter 3:
What Is Good Walking?

We walk every day across the house, around town, to our, cars and we don't realize that we have fallen into bad habits. Some people slouch. Some people get into the habit of carrying too many things (a big purse, an arm full of books or binders, tilting to the side when you carry groceries, etc.) and, thus, have altered their walking habits without realizing it.

While it doesn't seem like it, these bad habits could be hard on your walking regimen and could end up making a few hidden problems worse. Take a look at what good walking is so that you know you're doing this simple task in the correct way.

Keep your shoulders back. Kyphosis is a growing problem in the older generations. Kyphosis refers to the rounding of the upper back right about where your neck connects to the shoulder area, and it can sometimes give the appearance of someone having a hunchback, a slouching posture, leaning forward, or the body in a kind of downward sag.

While most of the time this happens due to osteoporosis, congenital disease, or cancer, you can prevent it happening to your future self by making sure that you don't slouch and that you keep your shoulders back while you walk. This activity helps to strengthen the shoulders and chest and to prevent them from becoming concave.

Keep your chin parallel to the ground. While "hold your head high" is often a euphemism for being confident (which we've already talked about as an element of walking), keeping your chin parallel to the ground while walking is beneficial beyond confidence.

Keeping your head high helps to keep your shoulders from sagging and from Kyphosis, and it also helps strengthen your neck muscles to create better posture. Additionally, you may find that while you're walking, other factors may be present that you need to be aware of. If you're walking in a gym on a treadmill, keeping your head up keeps you balanced and keeps you from falling off of the treadmill.

If you're walking in your neighborhood, keeping your head high keeps you alert to external factors out of your control, such as cars on the road, other people who are walking, loose dogs or wild animals, and it keeps your eyes on the goal ahead which helps to keep your set pace.

Hold in your stomach. There's a joke about how when someone's picture is about to be taken, someone might say, "Suck it in" or "Hold in your stomach." If, while you're walking, you pretend like someone is about to take your picture or if you're holding in your stomach to impress someone, you'll find that your overall health and wellness will be improved. Why? Because you're activating your stomach muscles, therefore you're engaging more muscles in the activity, and you'll not only burn more calories from that extra activity but you'll tone your stomach more. After a regular schedule of this, it may appear as though you are losing more weight in your middle area than you actually are because that area will be more toned and more controlled.

Select good footwear. It may seem obvious that you should have good shoes for walking, but it still deserves to be addressed. Have you ever found that you walk differently when you wear different shoes? People who wear flip flops walk differently than those who wear flat sneakers like Converse All Stars, and they all walk differently than someone who wears heels or someone who wears hiking shoes.

The best footwear for a walk is to wear running shoes. Even though you won't be running, running shoes provides the sufficient amount of ankle support and arch support that you will need to have an overall important posture. Shoes that are too flat on the bottom insole don't provide enough arch support and are, therefore, harder on your back and your leg muscles.

It's unlikely that anyone will be walking the neighborhood in heels, but these put unnecessary stress on the joints in the feet, particularly the toes. Even hiking boots aren't recommended (unless you're breaking them in for a hiking or backpacking trip) because running shoes provide the walker with more flexibility, and breathing space to the feet.

Application:

The next time you walk, start the walk off by keeping your shoulders back and your chin parallel to the ground. Hold in your stomach as you walk. Let your arms swing, but not independently—with control. These changes won't happen overnight for you, but see how often you focus on making these changes before they become habitual.

Chapter 4:
What To Eat Before And After You Walk?

If you're going to be holding in your stomach as you walk, it may not be the most comfortable thing for you to have eaten a gigantic breakfast before you take off. However, it's also not a good plan to eat nothing before you walk because you're going to be burning calories for weight loss and you don't want to get halfway into your walk and think that you might possibly pass out.

Additionally, it's important to hydrate before and after your walk, especially if you live near a desert or in a dry area, if you live in an area of high humidity, if you are walking in the summer or warmer months, or if you are walking while the sun is out. These and several other dietary concerns are part of what it means to eat right before and after your walk.

Before your walk

It's important to have a healthy snack before you walk. Because you should wait about three or four hours to work out after a heavy meal, a big breakfast before walking isn't a good idea. If you are a person who generally skips breakfast, have at least a big glass of water and a small cup of juice or a piece of fruit before you go.

Other great morning snacks include cereal, low-fat yogurt, a bagel, an English muffin, or a piece of fruit like an apple, a banana, or other fruits that you might prefer, depending on the season, such as peaches or cantaloupe. The best foods to eat before walking include foods with fluids because these also help to hydrate you.

If you are the kind of walker who prefers to walk after work or after dinner, vegetables are a great idea, and so are pasta and rice. Stay way away from fried foods, burgers, and soft drinks, as these don't contain enough of the right low-fat, low-fiber, fluid-rich components to optimize your walk.

After your walk

If you're walking for muscle toning, it's really important for you to have some kind of protein after your walk—generally within the first half hour of your walk. Kinds of protein could include hard boiled eggs, meats, beans, chocolate milk, or a protein shake. Don't go too crazy, though: your body only needs 10-20 grams of protein.

Long-distance

While long-distance walking is less of an everyday occurrence, you might decide to go on a long-distance walk after you've been walking for a while. If this is what you decide, start eating a lot of high-carb foods about 90 minutes before you start the walk, and make sure that during the walk you have plenty of water. A good rule of thumb for this kind of hydration is to plan on drinking two cups of water for every two hours of exercise.

Walk after meals

Recent studies have shown that walking 15 minutes after each meal for 15 minutes, or 45 minutes at the end of the day (still 15 minutes after that last meal) can help prevent diabetes. These studies suggest that walking after you eat slows or stops digestion and helps to use that calories that you've ingested toward the new activity instead of processing the food with normal (or sometimes elevated) levels of insulin. This can also help cut back on acid/esophageal reflux, as gravity is working the stomach acid down instead of sitting and allowing it to jump high where it normally burns. Studies suggest that walking 15 minutes after a meal can help cut acid reflux in half.

Hydration

While it has already been mentioned, hydration is extremely important before, during, and after your walk. If you're walking for only 15 minutes around the neighborhood, you don't need to take a water bottle with you, but it is important that you drink at least a large glass of water before you leave and a large glass of water after you come home. Nutritionists suggest that anytime you recognize that you are thirsty, you're already dehydrated, so if you find that you are thirsty; make sure that you continue to drink water until you feel full. You'll also find that the more water you drink, the less tempted you are to eat, which also helps reduce calories and, thus, lose weight.

Chapter 5:
How To Start Walking?

Okay, so we've talked about the health benefits of walking and how walking can improve your mindset and thus positively affect everything else in your life. We've talked about how to walk in good form. So now, how do you start walking? It's great to intellectually realize the benefits of walking and to intellectually commit to walking, but how do you integrate it into your schedule in an easy and stress-free manner? Here are a few tips:

Schedule

Remember how in the first chapter you jotted down a few ideas about a time in your schedule that would work for you? What are those times? Are you committing to every day or every other day? If you don't know yet, that's okay.

Physicians recommend that when you're starting out on a walking regimen, you should start by committing to three times a week, and then gradually increase it from there. You should always plan on at least one day off, and some personal trainers recommend that you shouldn't put your days off right next to each other or else it will be harder to get back after the break (thus, more tempted to lose the regimen entirely).

When you're first looking at your schedule, see if you try this:

> ➢ Monday on

> ➢ Tuesday off

> ➢ Wednesday on

➢ Thursday off

➢ Friday on

This gives you the weekend off to do other weekend-like activities without feeling like you have to incorporate an element of work. Even if you escalate to more days on and one day off, try to take Sundays off (if it works in your schedule). You need to have one day of a break in your schedule somewhere, and in our culture, Sundays are a celebrated day of relaxation.

Time of the day

You may have written in your journal about a certain time of the day that works best for you, and now is when you should consider when that is. Often professionals or other busy people will select the earliest time they can for walking. It helps as a kind of calm meditation before the day starts and gets crazy or out of control.

Some see it as a kind of grounding foundational time to get in touch with who they are. However, others prefer to walk in the afternoon when they get home from work or in the evening after dinner. Generally, the people that select this time of day view walking as a form of down-time, relaxation and de-stressing.

Other people might have other needs. For instance, a widow who has recently adopted a puppy may find that she needs to walk three times a day, including in the middle of the day to ensure that the puppy gets as much of an outlet for exercise as possible. If you are someone who has a puppy, has children, or has other needs that walking is related to, make sure that you budget your walk time appropriately to fit everyone's needs.

Just do it

Perhaps the best way to start walking is to just start walking. You can always adjust your schedule to something else if what you've started doesn't work, and you can always skip your walk one day if you have to for special circumstances like a business trip, a vacation, visiting family members, or any other scheduling hang-ups.

You can always start walking and realize later that you have bad posture and fix it. You can always take an extra day off if you have health problems that include you not walking on one day for whatever reason. But the important thing is to start walking. There will always be a reason why you shouldn't walk or that you don't feel like it today.

No one is going to walk for you except you. There are easy way to make walking work in your schedule, and there are harder ways, and only you are going to be the one to be able to see what works in your schedule with your lifestyle. Don't get hung up on excuses: while the walking schedule can be flexible, you still need to do it in order to get all of these fantastic health benefits.

Tip

If you wake up and "just don't feel like" walking, do it anyway. When you exercise, your body releases endorphins that make you feel better. Therefore, if you don't feel like walking before, you will feel glad about having walked later because chemically your body will tell you that it's glad it went. If you're sick, of course, that's something else entirely, but if you are in good health, trust that taking that step out of your door to start doing what is good for you will actually make you feel good, too.

Chapter 6:
Walking as an exercise

Now that you have understood walking is a basic habit, it is important to know that you need to walk enough to improve your health. It is suggested by most to take 10,000 steps each day for exercise; it is not just the count but the correct steps that has importance. Incorrect steps could tire your muscles and cause strain, which will have adverse effects on your body, thereby defeating the purpose of exercise.

Here are few tips which can take walking from a habit to an exercise.

Preparation

Picking out the right destination

Walking requires a proper well-spread, neat place. Ideal walking locations are naturally equipped with a flat terrain, clear path without any deviations, smooth surface and low vehicular traffic. Your neighborhood blocks are often a comfortable choice, but at times the road isn't what you're looking for or are comfortable with. In such a case, you will have to look out for walking in parks or other areas in your town.

Proper footwear is a must while walking, as there will be a lot of strain on your feet which could cause pain. Wear something that can handle the pressure as well as something that suits the weather, as comfort and quality are the main characteristics.

Drive your car to a park only if it is a necessity. Most parks are flat and have a calm ambience, and walking to a park will only boost your mind. If the city park isn't nearby, there are options of biking boulevards or paths on either sides of the road that are well-maintained and have minimal ups and downs. These can serve as good alternatives for walking as they have minimal traffic.

Shopping malls are good locations for walking as they are leveled, spun over huge areas, and have different paths. They also have few stores which keep you entertained if you have something on your mind. The crowd, though large in numbers, is dispersed and moving. The shoreline can be a calm and peaceful place for an early morning walk to get some air if you live near the beach or a large water body.

Employees who can't afford time can always use a treadmill as a source of their walking.

Picking out your music

Listening to music as you take a walk is extremely comforting if you are bored from staring at trees and other things you come across. It is suggested to listen to inspirational and pop music to help you focus on other parts of your life and maintain a good tempo. Think about your dinner last night; think about your favorite movie's plot, but do not deviate to something as dull as your work or as complicated as the purpose to life. Upbeat music will keep you walking with no stress. A walk is your chance to unwind and let loose!

Don't aim for the stars

If your body has been resting for a long period of time, starting slower and aiming for short laps is recommended. Monitor your progress by making short term goals and setting them down on paper. Walking is one of the basic exercises and hence does not need any form of stressful exertion. A fresh body with correct posture and equipment will be able to walk for a couple of hours. As it is a mild exercise, your body won't tire as much as it does for running or weightlifting exercises.

Be mentally strong

This is one of the key aspects and possibly one of the easiest ones, but will be extremely hard to capture once gone. Get your mind set for an investment as a slow and steady approach is required.

Be patient

Walking as an exercise is all about making efforts towards a better and healthier lifestyle, and it's a change for the long run—a whole lifetime. Using walking for one-shot fitness or for reducing weight instantly will not be effective and could easily backfire.

Drink a lot of water

Consume at least 8-16 ounces of water an hour before you are about to walk. Drink more if you plan to walk for a longer time or for a longer distance. Drinking extra will work as a reserve and you could avoid getting dehydrated mid-trek in the hot sun, which would be a devastating situation. Carrying a metal water bottle will be convenient and keep you hydrated throughout your trek as you walk.

We also suggest you not to drink too much water to the extent that your body can't process it immediately. Some people develop stomach cramps in this manner. Also, do know that there are minimal chances of finding a bathroom while on a long walk.

The walk

Walk in circles

Create a path in such a way that no matter how far you get from your starting point, you are able to get back to it. Walking in circles or an oval path for half a mile around is ideal. This way, you also minimize the chances of getting lost or losing your track while walking. If convenient, extend your walk past what you set for—raise the bar. Walking is lighter on your body than most exercises, so don't be afraid to go for it!

Time management

Time management is important for smooth flow of almost every activity. For walking, you need to fix the duration of your walk as per your convenience. Dedicate to a specific duration of time and be sure of accomplishing it. Do not worry about the length, think about the outcome. Just keep moving until you reach it. A 2-5 minute walk each day is a good start as you can increase the time on a weekly basis.

Try to avoid measuring the distance of how far you have walked. Faster and farther walks will come with experience.

Bettering your walk

Dedicate more time

Every day or week, increase your walking time by 30 seconds to 1 minute for as long as it is convenient or sustainable. The addition doesn't have to be consistent as long as a bare minimum is increased. Set the goal and measure your progress. After reaching 10 minutes, the rate of addition will not be exponential, but continue trying to increase your walking time slowly and steadily.

Add more speed

If your body can sustain 45 minutes of walking daily, try setting the bar higher and move from the oval tracks onto the city streets with faster legs. You will encounter inconsistent roads which will make the walk more challenging and then you could regulate your speed.

Continue to find more difficult tracks and you could possibly find the ultimate challenge of hiking up hills and cliffs.

Reach your target heart rate

For better accuracy and precision, you need to have a heart rate monitor and wear it during your walking. You can also measure it manually, it is the rate of exercise where your heart starts pumping faster and you start panting. If you are under your target heart rate (THR), you will need to increase your speed for the effectiveness of the exercise.

Your body will start burning accumulated fat only when you cross your THR for a sustained period of time. When it comes to a mild exercise like walking, weight loss and a healthy body will only be achievable through long durations of work and sweat, not just in a day or a week.

Experiment

After your body is accustomed to a general physical routine, try experimenting with your intervals. Walk at increased speeds for one to two minutes and then drop back to your normal rate for two minutes. Practice your interval training every day or alternate day, until you reach your desired total time which includes your rest times. As you become more physically fit, minimize your resting time until it is down to a minute or less. With this you can make sure that you walk normally when you're resting instead of coming to an abrupt stop.

Chapter 7: Walking workouts

In the previous chapter, we have looked at how walking can be implemented as an exercise. Now we will look at various walking workouts which can help us achieve a toned body. Whether you want to burn excess fat, increase your energy levels, motivate yourself, tone your body in a few places or just want to be physically fit, body workouts are necessary for you.

Make your fat burn

This could make you lose some fat and shrink down in a month by implementing vigorous and intense walks to your daily routine. You'll burn more amount of fat during and after your cardio workouts. There are also other options which align with your convenience like a 10-minute routine for busy weekdays and an indoor option for rainy weather and working professionals. For better results, a minimum of 20 minutes high-intensity walking (coupled with workouts and longer sessions to burn more) on three alternate days in a week is required. For other days of the week, do a mild or moderate activity for about 30 minutes.

Walking Workout 1: Treadmills

Time: 30 minutes

Treadmills are ideal for working professionals who need a toned body but have no time to walk around the city. With treadmills, there is no need to worry about weather, traffic or darkness. Tracking your speed increase as you become fit is also a huge motivator.

Walking Workout 2: Sprint

Time: 25 to 30 minutes

The faster you walk, the farther you can go and more fat is burned. Sprinting is capable of burning as many as 175 calories in one session. Calm your body down by a 5 minutes warm up, try walking as fast as you can for about 10 minutes. Keep in mind how much distance you have covered. Then turn around and walk back at a brisk pace, slowing down progressively. This way casual walking will rest your body. The next time you go, aim faster and farther than your previous attempt.

Walking Workout 3: Marathon

Time: 60+ minutes

Hour-plus workouts can reduce more than 5 times the amount of fat when compared with a 30-minute walk. Nearly 350 calories could be burnt during an hour long walking episode. This can help you walk in shape for events like a half marathon by providing you with an experience of longer strain. It can also be integrated with your social events, where you plan to meet up with friends and walk with them for a stretch of your route.

Walking Workout 4: For excess belly fat

Time: 10+ minutes

A high-intensity workout like this one is a belly-buster and can burn a considerable amount of belly fat. This can be ideal if you are looking to shape your abs or if you want to get a faint hint of them. Use the following tips for your walk:

Draw your stomach in towards your spine. Try to maintain the contraction, but don't hold your breath. This will help the muscles get shape.

Let your legs move freely, as one leg swings forward and back in such a fashion that the hip should move with the motion. This slight swivel of your hips makes your lower body rotate, stretching more stomach muscles to tighten at your belly.

Walking Workout 5: Bit of everything

Time: 10 minutes

Intense activities can be clubbed into a whole 10 minute workout and this is capable of burning 70% of the body fat. This workout is a time saver and is ideal for people on the go.

Warm up your body with slow-moderate walking for three minutes, walk at a brisk pace for the next minute and follow it up with 30 seconds of jogging. The jogging can be an on-the-spot jog or dynamic. For the next minute, walk quickly and follow it with jumping jacks activity for 30 seconds. Walk quickly for the next minute and follow it with side jumps for 30 seconds and continue your fast walk for one minute. Jog for 30 seconds and then calm your body down with slow and easy base for the last minute.

Recharge your body and mood

This routine can be used when you need to rev up your energy and brighten your mood. All you need is a 10 minute stroll for improved circulation which activates your mind. Extending it to 30 minutes could give you an 85% boost. These work as wake up calls and will work for 12 hours and recharge your body and mind for further activities of the day and achieve your goal. Be it to lose weight, tone your body or get healthy, this workout can help.

Walking Workout 6: Stress buster

Time: 10+ minutes

Revitalize your mind and body with this workout that is also known as a 'Happiness walk'. The longer and further you walk, the more benefits you'll see.

Step 1: Look at your feet, feel the blood flow to your feet. Feel the firm ground beneath you. Tap the ground and focus on holding awareness of your steps for 2 to 3 minutes.

Step 2: Breath in and out. Focus on it. Maintain an upright posture and expand your chest. As you inhale, think of all the energy you're taking in. Exhale the toxins of tiredness and pain. Feel the positive air stream into your lungs and your cells.

Step 3: Talk to yourself. You're your own critic and motivator. Thinking about the process of breathing will calm you down and increase your attention span.

Walking Workout 7: Brainpower Booster

Time: Under 20 minutes

This sort of workout can help the body assess its hand-eye coordination. It activates the brain and some of the underused muscles, such as your outer and inner thighs. This routine can be ideally done on an average school track of a quarter mile.

The workout:

Lap 1: In this lap, start at the beginning of the curved end of the track and walk at your warm up pace for one whole lap.

Lap 2: Here you need to turn sideways to the next track, so that your right leg is ahead. Shuffle around to the other part of the track and walk to the rear on a straight track. Shuffle sideways to the next bend with your left leg ahead and walk forward on the straight track.

Lap 3: Here you need to repeat the process done in lap 2, which was walking sideways and backward and then going sideways and towards the front

Lap 4: Here you need to walk ahead and slow down progressively for a whole lap. This would be a mile long walk, for a ¼ mile path. You can practice more sets and go on for half or even full sets of each type of walking.

Walking Workout 8: Host under trees

Time: 5+ minutes

Nature can make you feel happy and revitalize you in minutes. By exercising in a natural set up and prolonging it (a lunchtime park walk or an all-day mountain hike), you can improve on your memory and attention span more effectively than you can by walking in an urban city. That's because there are fewer distractions and it's much more relaxing.

Keeping your body firm

Addition of body toning exercises or techniques to your general daily routine can turn your morning walks into full-fledged muscle exercises. Aim for a specific tissue every week.

A specific workout can be done once or twice a week and the related lower-body and upper-body routines can be done on alternate days. Avoid working on the same tissue for consecutive days. For effective firming, do walking routines from other sections on in-between days to burn excess fat and get your muscles in shape.

Walking Workout 9: Walking poles

Time: 25 minutes

Usage of walking poles is known to boost your calorie burn by up to 46% as the workout involves the whole body movement, with proper angles of the hand and the shoulder. It gets your arms and core involved for all-round firming. The poles will reduce the shock impact on your joints.

Walking Workout 10: Treadmill Butt

Time: 25 minutes

The speed is maintained constant throughout the workout with a progressive incline. You can do the whole 25-minute routine or cut for the 5-minute hill climbs for a shorter session.

Walking Workout 11: Arm Shaper

Time: 20 minutes

Warm up your body for 4 minutes with easy walking. Raise the bar to moderate intensity and do the first exercise for 25 reps. When you're down, drape the resistance band around your neck and speed up for a quick walk similar to the one when we are in a hurry. Repeat the 25 reps for 20 minutes, until you've done all the exercises. Calm your body down with 4 minutes of easy walking. You can set the bar higher with more difficulty with the band, by placing hands closer together so you're using less band, or easier by separating hands for more slack.

Walking Workout 12: Butt Firmer

Time: 16+ minutes

Walking uphill burns about 25% extra muscle fibers due to faster signaling and firming as opposed to strolling on flat ground. This is because the body is under strain and the body strives forward. For better results, find a hill that takes 2 to 2½ minutes to climb and try this workout.

The workout: The workout is an outdoor challenge. Walk at slow pace for about 5 or 10 minutes as warm-up. Climb up and go down and follow it with 2 minutes of quick and brisk pacing on a flat surface. Repeat the steps and you'll achieve firmer and better-shaped butts. Finish with 5 minutes of strolling to cool down.

Walking Workout 13: Sculpt All Over

Time: 25 to 40 minutes

During this workout, you'll improve your strength moves for your walk and cardio plus toning.

The workout: Script out your strength moves on a paper. Use different exercises to practice on all important muscles, such as bench push-ups, tricep dips, lunges, walking planks, and power jumps. Drop them in a jar and draw them before a walk. Warm up at a slow-pace for 3 to 5 minutes, and then walk quickly for 5 to 10 minutes. Stop and do one of the strength moves for 10 reps. Continue with your quick walking for about 5 to 10 minutes, and follow it with your next strength move. Completing it for another cycle will be your final move. Calm your body for 5 to 10 minutes.

Walking Workout 14: Leg Toner

Time: 5 minutes

This workout is suggested as it has an easy home routine and can be done indoors. As it doesn't take much of your time, it can be done anywhere (need stairs) to tone your legs.

The workout:

1. Walk up and down one stair at a time as you would do usually.

2. Walk up sideways slowly, crossing your bottom foot over top and walk down by keeping your head up. You can also repeat this step by changing your orientation.

3. Step up, then go down on first stair level, start with your right foot and then move it in a motion of right up, left up, right down, left down for about 10 times. This can be repeated starting with your other foot too.

4. Skip a step while going up the stairs and then quickly come down by using each step.

5. Run up the stairs and brisk walk down the stairs.

6. Repeat steps 4 and 5 for four or five times.

7. At the bottom of the stairs, keep your right foot on the first or second step, bend your knees, and lower into a lunge. Your right knee directs the other nail to better

the signal. For a cycle, start with your right hand and then continue with your left leg and repeat the process.

8. Brisk walk up and down the stairs by stepping on each step precisely.

Chapter 8:
Maintenance

In the previous chapters, we have seen how walking affects our body and how we could use it for exercise and working out. As we increase the time span, staying true to a nutritious diet and regular exercise could seem like a taxing task, no matter how physically strong you are.

Especially during the holiday season, where there are instances of meeting with family and ample amounts of holiday goodies on the table, it is indeed the most difficult time to control your impulses. In this chapter, we explore how to stick to your diet and maintaining exercise throughout the year, especially during the holidays.

It is a fact that the typical American gains about 2 pounds during the holiday season, but most people never burn the fat they gain throughout the year, leading to an excess fat deposition in tissues over years it makes your body look bulgier.

You can never overcome the power of temptation, not completely, and most definitely not during the holiday season. However, you could stop yourself from eating unhealthy and junk food, which could make you gain more fat. You can achieve that by strengthening your mind and being mentally strong. Here are simple tips to get started:

Think ahead and plan accordingly, always

If you're attending a family dinner or an event, make sure to eat a high-protein snack right before leaving. The high protein in the snack won't just fill your stomach but will also make you feel less hungry when compared to a high-carbohydrate snack.

Think of healthier alternatives for your snacks to keep you from starving. This would be beneficial when you're on the go or in class. If you're hosting an event, search for healthier versions of holiday foods. This would benefit both you and your guests.

Avoid high calorie drinks

Liquid calories are as important a part of diet as are the calories you eat. Drinking carbonated soft drinks or sweetened sodas is not suggested as they have high carbohydrate content. Instead, drink water or a glass of red wine and other clear alcohols with club soda and a splash of lime. This way, you're having the same taste of a drink but are making a healthier choice.

Focus on something other than food

The holidays are about spending precious time with the people you love, celebrating the times you've spent together as memories. Spend time in doing activities that don't necessarily revolve around food. Be active in a group, try a new board game together, go for a walk in the park, or even take yoga classes together to make memories and photos which focus on the fun you had more than on what you ate.

Avoid binge eating

In this fast world, extra stress is a part of everyone's lives. It accompanies us almost everywhere, even to our beds. We all respond differently to stress, most of us turn to food for comfort, especially during the holidays where there's loads of it available. Keep stress away by dedicating at least 30 minutes for yourself every day, not matter how busy you are. Do self-motivating activities like going for walks, meditate, reading a book— anything you would enjoy.

Exercising is top priority

Avoid over-sleeping and skipping your morning workout because you are tired from the night before. This would ruin your mornings and your schedule. Instead, use exercise as motivation to wake up early and workout as you have nothing to lose. Challenge your body in daily situations and activities like taking the stairs, doing sit-ups during TV advertisement breaks, walking a little farther before taking a cab, cycling to get the groceries. Increase your heart rate from time to time and this will keep you fit and healthy consistently without doing much. This way you could skip a workout or two.

Sleep right

Staying up late and not getting enough sleep is one of the trademarks of attending social events. Unfortunately, reduced sleep hours can have a critical impact on you as sleep deprivation could lead to weight gain, lower immunity levels thereby making you more disease-prone. Set a strict bedtime and stick to it for a month. Pick and choose between important and not so important events that could keep you up later than usual and regulate your bedtime in a way wherein you have enough sleep.

Focus on these goals throughout the year and stay committed to stay healthy. These tips will help you avoid high calorie foods, focus on other activities and regulate your food intake. The next step is to maintain exercise and workout regularly.

Maintaining exercise

Unhealthy habits may not show immediate effects but long term consequences are very indicative and one cannot escape from them. There isn't a doubt we'd all like to change them, but that change often comes a little too late. For some, the most challenging part is finding the mental strength or determination to make those changes, while for most it's trying to regulate to new healthy habits. Exercising and healthy food habits are trickiest to habituate to.

You can get accustomed to your habits by understanding certain motives and barriers to your body. Maintaining a healthy habit is all about thinking straight. You need to:

1. Think about your motive to exercise. Remember, through a healthy and fit body you can make most disease causing organisms ineffective.

2. Identify what restricts you; what creates a barrier between you and a healthy you.

By understanding this, you're almost there, on the path to maintain your healthy habits and get fit. There are few common motivating factors for exercising like weight loss, general health, fitness and a presentable body structure. Common barriers are time, stress, work routine and laziness. Here are few tips to make exercise a part of your life.

There are a plenty of suggestions and tips that will help you maintain exercise as a habit:

Social support

Find someone who's close to you, like a friend, family member, coach or mentor, who will guide you through your effort to end some of your undesirable habits. If they could partner with you for exercise, you could motivate each other when the other doesn't feel like exercising and mutually benefit each other.

Make observations

Record your exercise time or the distance you have walked with various speeds. Through such analysis, you can set short-term and long-term goals, which can motivate you, especially after three or four weeks when you can see yourself improving and note how much you've progressed and how much more you could achieve.

Make no excuses

Avoid making excuses especially in the first month. It is a delicate phase where your body is adapting to the strain and any irregularities could have drastic consequences. Whenever you're tired, stroll and walk slowly for about 5 minutes. The hardest part is not to begin the journey but to maintain it.

Experiment

Inculcate fun activities like walking, cycling, swimming, tennis, weights, yoga, and gym classes into your workout. Do various such activities to avoid boredom.

Reward

Select a short-term goal and get there. On doing so, reward yourself appropriately and think progressively. Habits will develop when you positively reinforce them at specific times and on a regular basis into your lifestyle. Developing a habit is more about replacing unhealthy behaviors with more desirable routines.

Checkmarks

- ➤ First step towards change comes from within you.

- ➤ Behaviors can be learned only through repetition and reinforcement; commit yourself to the positive.

- ➤ Record yourself, analyze and better yourself wherever you possible.

- ➤ Find a family member, trainer or friend who you could bet with.

- ➤ Investing in your health and training could motivate you to jump start as you generally have nothing to lose.

Chapter 9:
Treadmill Practice

The treadmill was an amazing invention for its time. It was engineered by William Edward Staub, an English mechanical engineer. Although it was invented to serve as an object for punishment for slaves; modern technology and development of the human race has now made it a machine that offers a powerful workout.

It is under your control and you get to choose your own difficulty level, based on your fitness levels and abilities. The device serves as an alternative to running outside, if the conditions aren't suitable. During such scenarios, treadmill running is lighter on your body than outdoor running because you it's completely under your control and that doesn't give you much strain. A treadmill has various customizations, which helps it recreate outdoor running and tests our body's potential.

There are few key points that you have to keep in mind for this practice, especially when you want to track your treadmill sessions for length, frequency and intensity. You can then figure out how you could experiment and add variety to your practice to avoid boredom. Plan out your goals, something that challenges you, makes you struggle and sweat-yet at the same time is achievable without support.

- ➢ Things to expect: Boost in energy levels

- ➢ Difficulty level: Anything that challenges you

- ➢ Time: A minimum of 30 minutes

Getting Started

1. Plan out the length and intensity of your treadmill runs

2. Extreme and casual workouts

3. Figure out how to add spice to your sessions and know when to stop experimenting

4. Make a schedule of your workout with adequate rest hours

5. Get your body ready for a workout both physically and mentally, before and after each workout

6. Note down observations and have record

Note:

- You might want to consider buying your own treadmill

- Use good pace

- Get additional help from a physiologist

Plan out the length and intensity of your treadmill runs

Length of workout

The length of your workout depends on how well you can manage your time. National Institutes of Health has set a 30 minute workout period for 5 times a week as a recommended standard for young individuals. You can vary your workout length as per your daily body practice and intensity for each session.

Workout Duration

Calculate the number of calories your body needs to take in to function properly. This way you can determine how many calories are needed to stabilize your current weight and eventually how many to lose weight. There is an optimal number of calorie intake, which varies with age, activity and whether you aim to lose, maintain or gain weight. Knowing your Basal Metabolic Rate (BMR) can also help you analyze about how much exercise your body can handle.

Intensity

It's not just about running, it's about running with speed (pace) or with incline (grade). Aim at medium to high intensity and track your exercise intensity by interpreting the strain you need to take for your desired target.

Extreme and casual workouts

Speed

Walking, jogging and running are all helpful workouts but most of us do not integrate them in one session. Working out is all about bettering yourself. Take it slow early on with your walk and gradually line it up to a jog with few runs in there. Generalized speed has been set for certain activities; you could always vary your speed as per your liking:

- ➢ 3.5 For Walking

- ➢ 5.0 For Jogging

- ➢ 6.0 For Running

- ➢ 9.0+ For a Sprint

Incline

The treadmill is a device that simulates an ideal track for running, which is easier than outdoor running. Set the treadmill at a 1% incline to feel a resistance similar to outdoor running.

Advantages

As incline increases your heart beat at a slower walking pace, there is less impact on knees and hips. Helps you keep your spine erect, which increases your speed. It stretches Achilles tendons and the calves.

An incline is similar to hiking. Walking at 3 mph could seem a slow pace but it's very grueling as a sustained pace at 15% incline without any assistance. There is increased motion at the lower body, which is crucial for body development. Slow walking on an incline is a very good challenge, set a pace and incline that are suitable for you depending on your body's fitness levels.

Basic Treadmill Workout - Walking Hills

A 5 minute warm up, either level or with incline is essential before a workout.

Find your customized setting, which challenges you by varying speed and incline yet is manageable enough to sustain for 30 minutes without collapsing. If you're new to the workout, your calves will tire down before your lungs do.

Throughout the workout, experiment with the protocol by doing faster walks at low inclines and very slow walks at higher inclines.

When to stop experimenting

Activity variety

The treadmill gives you a chance to buildup from slow walking to a run. You can also consider adding breaks in your workout session where you vary your workout intensity. Design a custom workout program for yourself or use one of the inbuilt programs to find a workout that suits your needs.

Intervals

Interval workouts have changes in speed and incline spread well to burn more calories, adapt and keep you focused. The workout is based on shift up in heartbeat during the intensity changes and holds a static state for about 5 minutes. The interval you choose is one that will bring you to high stress levels with a resting phase to catch your breath.

Basic Interval Workout Tips

The speeds and inclines recommended are only provided for a standard workout. You can go faster, slower, higher or lower and vary it as per your fitness level. These intervals can last anywhere between 30 seconds to 10 minutes.

The shorter the interval, the higher the intensity levels, which could sustain only for short times. This way, for a one-minute interval you should feel out of breath after one minute. The recovery intervals are calm and relaxed enough for you to catch your breath. These last over a minute to 5 minutes.

Some treadmills have integrated interval programs, but vary with model for the incline changes, not the speed. The incline range is limited for most models. For example, if you want both very high and low inclines in one program, and set it for experimentation there will be only a 6 percent change. There is no necessity of a program offering both very high and low grades.

Manual adjustment is recommended and is most accurate. Have repeat intervals set for 3 to 10 times depending on the workout duration.

Follow a schedule

Frequency

Based on the duration of your workout, strain and other exercises you will do, you can determine how often you would want to run on the treadmill.

Schedule it

After assembling your data, schedule your workout. Making a timetable for your workouts will help you in your performance as you are more likely to get habituated to it. The main goal of exercise timetable is to maintain it, so schedule at least 4-5 sessions, don't skip any and you will make it a habit. Remember to have a day or two for you and your family, resting and socializing have equal shares in your schedule.

Get your body ready

Warm up prior to each work out

A warm up is crucial for the body to avoid injuries from the strain. The objective of the warm-up is to raise the temperature of the entire body preparing it for strenuous activity.

Cool down following each workout

Cool down after a workout session is just as important as the exercises. The primary objective is to gradually decrease the intensity of the aerobic activity and return to a state of rest.

The cooling down plays a major role by,

- Preventing blood pooling, returning the blood back to the heart than allowing it to pool in the muscles which causes spasms

- Gradually bringing the heart rate back down to a normal beat

- Ensuring that the brain continues to receive a sufficient supply of blood and oxygen and breathe out properly.

- Preventing lactic acid accumulation in muscles.

Maintain a record

Track your activity, duration, intensity and response times. You might want to consider buying your own treadmill

Buying your own treadmill would save time and you would not have to rely on going to the gym for maintaining exercise.

Using good pace

Apart from the vigorous exercises, it is vital for your body to maintain proper form when using a treadmill. This way you absorb all the benefits from the exercise as well as stabilize your form.

Look Ahead

Look and keep your eyes on the ground about 10-20 feet ahead of you. Maintain a straight and erect posture. Keep your head high, spine straight and shoulders raised. Keep your shoulders relaxed and symmetrical but do not hunch.

Place your hands on your waist and slowly relax. The arms are to be inclined at a 90-degree angle and positioned to just touch your hip.

Have a short stride, which helps in minimizing the impact on your legs. Stamp a mid-foot strike and avoid heel striking. This could send a shock to the sensitive nerves around your legs.

Don't hold the handrails

Holding the treadmill rails will force you to hunch over; this could soon lead to neck, shoulder, and back pain. It is an ineffective form of running though you may feel faster, but in reality, you're risking impact of your load on your legs and making it easier by pulling yourself.

Outside running does not have any rails, try to mock such conditions. If you are falling 'down', you're at a fast pace or a high incline. Do not underestimate yourself, the railing is only for support and is essential only for beginners. Cheating your workout by touching the rail might seem easy but is an addictive habit once caught. You can always slow down than cheat yourselves.

Chapter 10:
Rules for a Runner's Diet

In this chapter we review six rules designed for a runner's diet.

Most of the runner's eating plans have no real food in them, not that they're starving but they consume a lot of calories in the form of nutrient-enhanced drinks, energy bars, and zero-fat products. They usually miss out on the vegetables, fruits, lean meats, whole grains, which are better than packaged products.

There's more to food than just nutrients. In our system, vitamins, minerals, and other essential nutrients are associated with several other molecules such as color components in fruits and vegetables, fibers and essential fats in seeds, nuts, and dairy foods. Consuming a whole fruit or vegetable is a whole package of necessary elements required for growth and development.

High-energy protein bars and drinks is an alternative way to get the bare minimum required nutrients for runners. Consuming them through rich food is regulated and advantageous. Follow these six rules daily will give your body all it needs, in excess to running and exercising in full swing.

Seed-oriented foods

Seeds are often discarded or have lesser priorities but most of the seeds (whole grains, beans and tree nuts) contain an all important combination of nutrients necessary to give life, which means they consist of health-boosting compounds. Apart from necessary proteins and fats, seeds contain bio-active antioxidant species like phenolic compounds and ferulic acid.

According to research, a dietary plan with plant seeds can improve health and optimize body weight. People who eat whole grains and beans have minimal risk of type 2 diabetes and develop cancer. They also have low cholesterol levels. The following seed-oriented dish is ideal for people who need to be on their feet 24x7.

Walnut and Blueberry Bran Pancakes

Ingredients

- 1 1/2 cups whole milk

- 1 cup instant oats

- 3/4 cup sifted all-purpose flour

- 1/2 cup walnuts, chopped

- 3/4 cup blueberries

- 1/4 cup oat flour

- 1 tablespoon baking powder

- 2 tablespoons honey

- Salt

- 2 eggs, beaten

Method

1. Take a bowl and add oats, flour, baking powder and salt. Whisk.

2. Add milk and eggs, whisk for a couple of minutes.

3. Mix honey to the batter and combine well.

4. Add walnuts and blueberries and mix thoroughly.

5. Pour out a ladle on a hot greased pan.

6. Cook till the top looks bubbly. Flip.

7. Cook properly on the other side too and serve in a plate.

Fruits and veggies

As we already know, eating fruits and vegetables supplies your body with vitamins and carbohydrates for your daily functioning. They also have few calories, which can stabilize your weight. More importantly, the color of the fruit or vegetable like yellow, orange, red, green, purple etc plays a major role. There are several pigments that apart from imparting color offer health benefits.

The pinkish red in pomegranate is the anthocyanins pigment, the deep red in tomatoes is the lycopene pigment, and the bright orange in carrot comes from beta-carotene. Pigments like these can lower your risk of cancer, heart disease, and Alzheimer's, while having a positive effect on your memory. They can also help minimize inflammation caused by disease or heavy exercise as they are antioxidants.

Eating a variety of colorful foods will be advantageous as all these pigments need to be present and associate with each other to give a positive result. This explains why only consuming beta-carotene in supplements doesn't lead to the same health improvements as eating the whole palette of colors would. The following dish has all the essential pigments associated together.

Grilled Vegetable with Key Lime Chimichurri

Ingredients

- 3 bell peppers, all colors, chopped

- 2 mushrooms, quartered

- 2 zucchini, sliced into rounds

- 1 onion, diced

Vegetable Rub

- freshly ground black pepper

- 1 tablespoon dried orange rind

- Salt

- 1 teaspoon sea salt

- Chili powder

Green Sauce

- 3 bay leaves, dried

- 6 garlic cloves, crushed

- 1 fresh Poblano pepper, chopped

- 1 fresh Serrano chili, chopped

- Sea Salt

- 1/3 cup parsley, finely chopped

- 3 key limes

- 1/4 cup fresh oregano, finely chopped

- 1/2 cup basil, finely chopped

- 1/3 cup olive oil

Method

1. Marinate the vegetables with the rub and keep aside.

2. Preheat the grill at 250 degrees Fahrenheit.

3. In a mortar add garlic, pepper, bay leaves, lime juice and salt and make a smooth paste. You can use blender as well.

4. In a mixing bowl add the above paste and all the herbs. Mix well.

5. Add olive oil to the bowl and whisk till it is combined thoroughly.

6. Skewer the veggies and grill properly.

7. Place the veggies with cooked wild rice and drizzle the sauce over it.

Drop the peeler

Eat plant foods with their skins intact. Almost all fruits and vegetables have outer skins as protective layer to shield them from UV light radiation, parasites, and other pathogens. Scientifically they are bursting with a vast range of phytochemicals, which can also improve your health. For example, grape skins have high amounts of resveratrol, and onion skins have quercetin, these compounds can help minimize heart disease risks, colon and prostate cancer chances, and strengthen your body.

The skin is rich in starch and fibers; they promote the growth of healthy bacteria in the intestinal tracts thereby relieving constipation and minimizing hemorrhoid chances. They improve intestinal functions, which assists in weight regulation. According to research, vegetable and fruit skin soluble and insoluble fibers blocks absorption of minor part of calories consumed on a high-fiber diet. This way eating fibers indirectly lowers body-fat levels while eating healthy. The following dish is rich in pigments and fibers, which could help in weight control.

Curried Lentils and Butternut Squash

Ingredients

- 1 cup dry mix lentils

- Whole Butternut squash

- 1 teaspoon chili powder

- 1 tablespoon olive oil

- 1 teaspoon ginger (grated)

- 1 tablespoon curry powder

- Salt

- Pepper

- 1/4 cup shredded coconut

Method

1. Take a baking tray and grease it properly. Keep aside.

2. Take a deep pot and put in the lentils in it. Cover with cold water.

3. Put the above pot over medium heat and let it boil. As it comes to a boil add chunks of squash.

4. Simmer till the squash gets soft.

5. Remove from heat, drain and keep aside.

6. Take out the squash chunks and, mash them properly.

7. Keep the oven on pre-heating mode at 400 degrees Fahrenheit

8. Take a large mixing bowl and add the lentils and squash. Mix.

9. Add olive oil with the spices to this. Add salt and combine well.

10. Ladle this out on the greased baking tray

11. Bake for 20 minutes or till done.

12. Serve with coconut sprinkled over.

Glass of milk

Milk products are a major part of a runner's diet, whether from a cow, a goat or even mammal milk (as opposed to soy milk) and others like cheese, yogurt, and kefir. Milk supplies calcium, a molecule which serves as a backbone for bone formation and strengthening of bones. Correct alignment and structure of bones is crucial for a runner.

Dairy food supplies a runner's muscles with an ample amount of protein to help adjust with the impact. Whey protein (protein found in dairy foods) can help strengthen one's immunity. Most milk products contain stearic acid, which can lower blood-cholesterol levels. Studies show that regular dairy consumption can lower your blood pressure. People who consume dairy in their diet tend to lose more fat than those who cut out on calories.

Fermented dairy products like yogurt, kefir, contains live bacteria, which help in digestion also boost immunity. Conjugated linolenic acid (CLA), a unique essential fat in dairy associated with bacteria can prevent constipation, reduce the pain of certain intestinal problems such as inflammatory bowel disease, and minimize episodes of yeast infections in women. For lactose intolerant people regular and regulated consumption of cultured dairy products can improve symptoms. The following recipe has ample amounts of dairy products and can offer your body with all the benefits mentioned above.

Seasonal Fruit Smoothie

Ingredients

- 1/2 cup seasonal fruits

- 3/4 cup low-fat yogurt

- 1 cup milk

- handful of Almonds

- Honey

Method

1. Peel the seasonal fruit (mango, peach, banana etc) and dice it.

2. Put this in a blender and add all the ingredients one by one.

3. Blend till smooth.

4. Pour out in a tall glass. Add ice or frozen fruit according to your taste.

Sea food

Eating cold water fish and other seafood provide a collaboration of almost all nutrients required for runners. A lot of seafood is a rich source of high energy protein and zinc, copper, and chromium– minerals, which are key elements in a runner's diet. Apart from all of this, the omega-3 fats found in fish make it a must have in a healthy person's diet.

According to research, people who eat fish and other seafood often have lesser risk of heart failure, vascular disease, and stroke. Fish intake also has psychological value, as it helps in reducing depression levels.

Recent studies have shown that low intake of fish, particularly the omega-3 fats has been associated with attention deficit hyperactivity disorder (ADHD) in children. Anthropological research has shown that our ancestors had more omega-3 fat consumption in their diet than we currently do.

This can easily be linked to our modern-day ailments, such as heart disease and Alzheimer's. The omega-3s in fish also have anti-inflammatory capabilities and help psoriasis and soreness in the muscles. The following seafood dish is tasty and a rich source of omega-3.

Spicy Salmon Lettuce

Ingredients

- 5 4-ounce salmon fillets

- 2 tablespoons olive oil

- Lime juice

- 1 tablespoon chili powder

- 1 teaspoon cayenne pepper

- 1 tablespoon cumin

- Salt

- Pepper

- 1 head butter lettuce

- 1 head radicchio

- 1 onion, diced

- 1 tomato, diced

- 1/2 cup prepared tzatziki

- 1/4 cup scallions, diced

Method

1. Keep the oven or grill on preheat mode at 400 degree Fahrenheit.

2. Grease a baking tray and add olive oil, lime juice and spices in it.

3. Add the fillets to this and coat them properly.

4. Marinate for 10 minutes.

5. Form cups of lettuce and radicchio by tearing them with your hand. Put the radicchio cups in the lettuce ones.

6. Brush the fillets with olive oil before putting them in the oven or grill. Cook until done.

7. Put the fish in the cups and add the tomatoes and the onions.

8. Drizzle tzatziki.

9. Garnish with scallions and serve hot.

Egg and meat

Eat meat, poultry, or eggs from free-range or grass-fed animals. By eating these along with dairy products, runners will easily cover their protein needs as these are rich sources of energy. They are a key source of iron and zinc, which is an important molecule for maintaining the red blood cells. These two minerals are easily absorbed by the body in the form of animal meat than through other supplement sources.

A vegetarian lifestyle is equally healthy, but studies do point towards the diet balanced with fruits, vegetables, whole grains, and thin cuts of meat like beef and skinless poultry. These foods help lower blood-cholesterol levels, stabilize blood pressure, and minimize heart failure risks.

Sticking to lean meats is very important, so meat from animals raised in open pastures that graze on grass is preferred than stockyard-raised, corn-fed, free-range meat. Grass-fed animal meat contains higher quantities of omega-3 fats and less blood vessel blocking saturated fats due to their healthier diets and higher activity levels.

The following dish is one such perfect meat dish, which does have compounds that clog your veins.

Cinnamon Chicken

Ingredients

- 1 chicken, cut into eight pieces

- 1 teaspoon ground cinnamon

- Salt

- Ground black pepper

- 5 garlic cloves, minced

- 2 onions, chopped

- 1 1/2 tablespoons extra virgin olive oil

- 1/2 cup dry white wine

- 1 cup chicken stock

- 1 cup water

- 1 6-ounce can tomato paste

- 1 tablespoon oregano, chopped

Method

1. Take a pan and boil water with some sea salt on medium heat. Keep aside.

2. Clean the chicken properly and pat dry with paper towels.

3. In a bowl add salt, cinnamon and pepper. Mix well.

4. Rub the above mixture over the chicken pieces. Coat it well and keep aside.

5. Crush three cloves of garlic.

6. Take a large skillet and heat it on high heat, reduce heat and add olive oil.

7. As olive oil heats, add the chicken. Brown the chicken for five minutes all over. Take out the chicken.

8. Add the onions and garlic to the pan. Cook for a couple of minutes. Stir constantly.

9. As onions turn golden brown in color, add wine.

10. When the wine evaporates, add chicken stock, water, oregano, tomato paste and the leftover garlic and mix well.

11. Add the chicken back to the pan and lower the flame. Add salt and pepper.

12. Cook for an hour till the chicken is tender.

13. Serve hot with rice or quinoa.

Conclusion

The best way to start walking is to start walking.

Walking is something simple that mostly everyone does something that we often don't think about it as an activity that we're already doing that we could embrace as a weight loss regime. Walking is something that we already do that we don't think is something we can focus on to produce confidence, control, mediation, peace of mind, and relaxation in a way that helps to improve weight loss, a healthy lifestyle, and a number of health benefits such as low blood pressure, preventing diabetes, preventing heart disease, and reducing acid reflux.

There are a number of ways to encompass good walking habits, and all of them can be adapted or improved upon as you walk through your workout regimen. Sometimes walking is good in the morning as a solitary activity that provides mediation and grounds you before the day gets crazy, and sometimes walking can be a communal activity as you bond with your new dog, as you walk with your family members, or as you get out in your neighborhood to meet the people you live around.

Walking is healthy activity that helps you to find order in your life. Control breeds confidence. Through walking you have the ability to control your schedule and to bring order to your easy and healthy workout regimen. At the very least, you can have control in your lifestyle by keeping at bay some health problems that you may have or may have the potential to have.

Walking provides a number of health benefits that make this activity important to integrate into your lifestyle. Don't just walk, walk for your body, walk for exercising and indulge in walking workouts. This way you won't just keep yourself fit but will tone down your body size and get in good shape.

Focus on long term results more, as maintaining a fit body throughout your lifetime is a challenge and something for others to envy about.

Eat at regular intervals of time and eat healthy. Step up and take walking to another level, running. This will keep your body in good shape for life.

Thank you again for downloading this book!

I hope this book was able to help you to start living your life as you should.

The next step is to apply what you've learned on a daily basis.

Finally, if you enjoyed this book, please take the time to share your thoughts and post a review on Amazon. It'd be greatly appreciated!

Thank you and good luck!

www.ingramcontent.com/pod-product-compliance
Lightning Source LLC
Chambersburg PA
CBHW070610290526
45790CB00002B/853